Toothache Relief Naturally

Home Remedies to Eliminate and Prevent Tooth Pain

The Alternative Healing Series

Hayden Anderson

This book is dedicated to anyone who is need of instant relief from tooth pain.

Copyright Act of 1976, the scanning, uploading and electronic sharing of any part of this book without the explicit written consent or permission of the publisher constitutes unlawful piracy and the theft of intellectual property.

If you would like to use material or content from this book (other than for review purposes), prior written permission must be obtained from the publisher.

You can contact the publishing company at admin@speedypublishing.com. Thank you for not infringing on the author's rights.

Speedy Publishing LLC (c) 2014
40 E. Main St., #1156
Newark, DE 19711
www.speedypublishing.co

Ordering Information:
Quantity sales; Special discounts are available on quantity purchases by corporations, associations, and others. For details, contact the "Special Sales Department" at the address above.

This is a reprint book.

Manufactured in the United States of America

TABLE OF CONTENTS

PUBLISHER'S NOTES i

CHAPTER 1: TOOTHACHE PAIN 1

CHAPTER 2: WHAT ARE THE CAUSES OF A TOOTHACHE? 3

CHAPTER 3: WHAT ARE THE SYMPTOMS OF A TOOTHACHE 9

CHAPTER 4: TOOTHACHE PAIN AND WHAT IT MEANS 11

CHAPTER 5: GET RID OF A TOOTHACHE WITH HOME REMEDIES 13

CHAPTER 6: TOOTHACHE PREVENTION 30

CHAPTER 7: CONCLUSION 34

MEET THE AUTHOR 36

MORE BOOKS BY HAYDEN ANDERSON 38

Publisher's Notes

Disclaimer

This publication is intended to provide helpful and informative material. It is not intended to diagnose, treat, cure, or prevent any health problem or condition, nor is intended to replace the advice of a physician. No action should be taken solely on the contents of this book. Always consult your physician or qualified health-care professional on any matters regarding your health and before adopting any suggestions in this book or drawing inferences from it.

The author and publisher specifically disclaim all responsibility for any liability, loss or risk, personal or otherwise, which is incurred as a consequence, directly or indirectly, from the use or application of any contents of this book.

Any and all product names referenced within this book are the trademarks of their respective owners. None of these owners have sponsored, authorized, endorsed, or approved this book.

Always read all information provided by the manufacturers' product labels before using their products. The author and publisher are not responsible for claims made by manufacturers.

Chapter 1: Toothache Pain

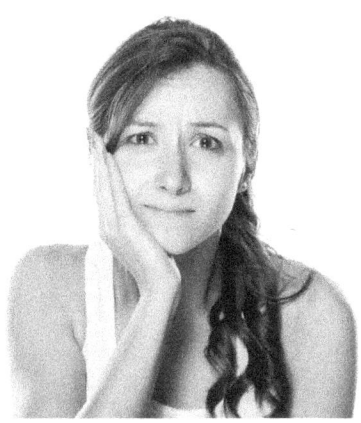

What is toothache pain? Seems like a straightforward answer doesn't it?, but it's one of those things where until you actually experience it firsthand for yourself nobody on the planet can ever explain it to you, no description is apt enough to detail the pain of a toothache until you yourself feel the intense shock of electricity permeate your tooth for the first time or the throbbing wave of pain that radiates from your jawbone that won't let up and for some reason seems to throb in time with your heartbeat.

A toothache can make your life a complete misery and it can bring grown men to their knees and until you do something about it it's nearly impossible to get on with your life. Eating and sleeping are difficult and so your health as a result deteriorates, not to mention the symptoms of the toothache itself could be an indication of more serious problems such as infection. The different types of toothache pain can also be an indicator of different problems that will be covered.

TOOTHACHE RELIEF NATURALLY

Technically a toothache is the pain in the tooth or teeth and around the jaw. It can be as described above as acute pain which is the intense, electrical jolt that stops you in your tracks or the more chronic throbbing that tends to linger.

Chapter 2: What are the Causes of a Toothache?

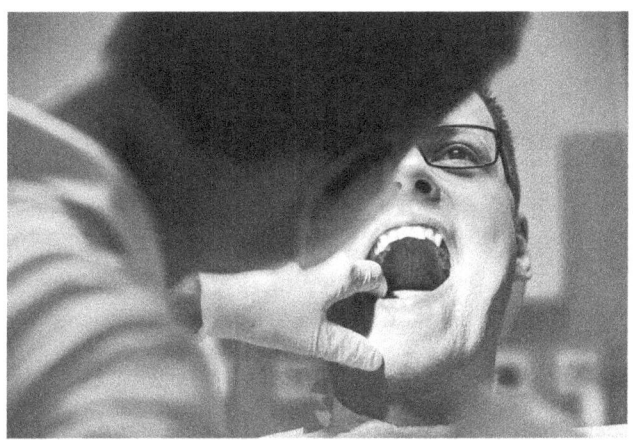

There could be several factors at play where the pain of the tooth itself is merely a manifestation of some other underlying issue. You don't appreciate it at this moment but your teeth are your body's warning system that something is wrong.

This can range from something as simple as hypersensitivity in teeth which cause them to react strongly to hot or cold liquids but with hypersensitivity it can even cause teeth to react strongly to cold drafts or excess dampness or moisture in the air.

Over forty million adults in the US alone (it's estimated that this proportion applies to the general population) suffer from tooth sensitivity due in part to the poor diet of our day. If you find your teeth becoming increasing reactive to hot and cold liquids and foods then it's a good chance you have sensitive or hypersensitive teeth.

This can also be an after effect of the tooth whitening process as the chemical bleach preparation applied to the teeth is acidic and weakens the protective tooth enamel layer increasing the risk of tooth decay and demineralization. This is why so many people feel that their teeth became noticeably more sensitive and brittle after whitening.

Most off the shelf brand tooth whiteners, particularly those contained in toothpaste don't actually whiten the teeth but actually irritate the gums making them a darker red. This gives the illusion of the teeth being whiter when in actual fact they are not.

For tooth sensitivity there are recommended toothpaste brands which can combat the symptoms of hypersensitivity while avoiding things like ice cream and hot drinks is recommended.

Another type of toothache is caused from excess wear on the teeth which can be accelerated by a condition known as "Bruxism", unconscious tooth grinding. Most people don't even know they have Bruxism as it tends to occur when the person is asleep. This constant grinding can wear the teeth down which leaves little separation between the dentine and the pulp. Once the dentine is exposed the pulp transmits messages of pain to the nerve hence the reason why dental cavities and cracked, injured teeth exposed to air and microbes are painful and sensitive.

Tooth sensitivity also occurs when gum recession takes place, the less protective gum layer covering the dentine and nerves the more teeth start reacting with time toward hot and cold foods and drinks.

Other causes of toothache are the more obvious culprits such as a cracked tooth, filling or veneer, dental caries from eating acidic, sweet foods that corrode the fillings and the tooth's protective enamel layer. This corrosion is caused from the bacteria that are present on the teeth which break down the sugary, refined food you eat and then excrete them in the forms of acids which then eats away at the protective enamel of the tooth causing a cavity, infection and eventually toothache.

Toothaches can also occur if the root is exposed to air and food or if you have sinus problems, that feeling of excess pressure in your head can manifest symptoms of sore, achy teeth.

If you have a cold or the flu or are feeling just generally run down you can feel it in your teeth. This is because the ears, nose and throat are all interconnected and impact one another even having a headache or extra tension around the head and facial muscles can create what resembles a toothache but really is a symptom of the tension itself. In this scenario, Tylenol or plain Aspirin would be the best solution for pain relief.

Another thing that exacerbates tooth pain is Gingivitis. Gingivitis causes gum line recession as tartar builds around the teeth in the absence of proper brushing and flossing. You can probably spot the early signs of Gingivitis such as red, inflamed, swollen gums that bleed easily when brushed or flossed.

Gingivitis starts out harmless enough as regular plaque but when allowed to build and accumulate for longer periods of time hardens into a yellow-brownish calcified cement-like structure which clings to the base of the teeth between the tooth and the gum line and becomes difficult to remove without the aid of a dentist. This hardened tartar must be physically scraped from the teeth.

The reason why tartar is such a problem is because when left untouched it pushes the gum line down causing it to recede exposing more tooth (hence the expression "long in the tooth"), in fact it is this that is responsible for the majority of tooth loss in adults rather than the cavities themselves.

The leading cause of tooth loss in American adults over the age of thirty-five is poor gum health (periodontal disease), staggeringly it is estimated that a massive seventy-five percent of this group have some form of gum disease and that sixty percent knew nothing about proper dental care with thirty-nine percent not attending the dentist regularly.

It's no wonder why people experience tooth loss and tooth related ailments more now than ever before due to poor diet from high sugar, refined foods, stressful lifestyle and the lack of education of proper dental hygiene.

We under estimate just how important our gums are because it's the gums that hold the teeth firmly in place acting as a support anchor to keep teeth in their socket, once tartar takes hold it shrinks the gums causing them to recede and pull back from the teeth, food gets into the little pockets as a result of the gum shrinkage. The lodged food attracts bacteria causing infection deep within the gum line, this in turn eats away at and shrinks the surrounding bone mass which is needed to firmly anchor the tooth.

This is what causes the teeth to become loose, if left untreated tooth loss eventually follows. Unless blunt force trauma occurs, tooth loss is a very gradual process over time where intervention can prevent the condition from worsening.

While the process of gum shrinkage occurs more and more, your tooth begins to become exposed where gum used to be making those now exposed areas more sensitive to hot and cold. It's because the more the gum line recedes that the more sensitive the tooth becomes as it gets closer to the tooth root. That is why so many adults are surprised at how sensitive their teeth became with age simply with the recession of their gums. Prevention in this case is the best solution but you can also halt the process with proper brushing, changing your toothbrush every three to six months and by only purchasing a medium hardness.

Believe it or not using a hard bristle toothbrush has been known to accelerate gum recession as it physically pushes the gums back when brushing with this type of toothbrush.

Flossing also helps get rid of the tartar forming plaque that settles below the gum line. Left untreated this contributes to gum disease, abscess and infection. If infection is left too long it can become dangerously toxic to the blood, the treatment to combat the problem would require a course of antibiotics.

Regular dentist visits ensures that any tartar build up is removed before it becomes a huge issue for your teeth in the future. It's such a gradual process that people too often don't pay attention to it, they put off going to the dentist because their teeth for now feel fine. Its' not until you're slapped with a nasty toothache that you realize it wasn't a problem that happened overnight but gradually accumulated over time.

So don't put off your regular dentist checks because early prevention is the best solution. Despite what you think gum recession doesn't have to be something that happens with age either, we have the technology to keep our teeth for life so early tooth loss should be a thing of the past.

There are technological developments in dentistry where you can actually have gum (soft tissue) grafts to reverse the effects of gum recession to recover previously exposed teeth. This type of surgical procedure is expensive, you must have a certain amount of gum tissue present in order to graft, requires a certain amount of healing time and not everyone is a candidate, for example diabetics area high risk factor and may not be suitable for this type of procedure. The best thing is to take preventative measures as soon as you can, the earlier the better.

While tooth loss is traumatic to experience itself, a more serious result of having Gingivitis and tartar build up is that it is a precursor to heart disease. What grows on your teeth indicates the bigger picture of what goes on within the body.

If you think about it we really are what we eat and what passes through our lips makes its way through our body. Doctors have proven that if you have a high accumulation and build up of tartar on the teeth then there is a high probability that this same calcified plaque attached to your teeth is also clinging to the walls of your arteries. This represents a bigger problem as this is the type of plaque build that causes high blood pressure, heart attack and stroke.

Angina (enlarged heart) can express itself as a painful jaw or toothache and your situation may be more medical than dental, your dentist may refer you to your doctor to get the appropriate treatment. Sometimes the onslaught of a heart attack can manifest itself as a pain on the left side of the jaw.

An aching and tenderness in the jaw hinge or both the jaw and cheekbones and the inside the ears, or the inability to chew properly may indicate the beginnings of the condition TMJ (Temporomandibular Joint disorder). This is where the joint responsible for smooth movement between the between the upper and lower jaws starts to wear making it difficult to eat, talk or yawn and can be very painful, especially after a night of tooth grinding.

So as you can see, tooth pain is not all bad, it can help warn us of more serious issues that we can get early detection and treatment of.

Chapter 3: What Are the Symptoms of a Toothache

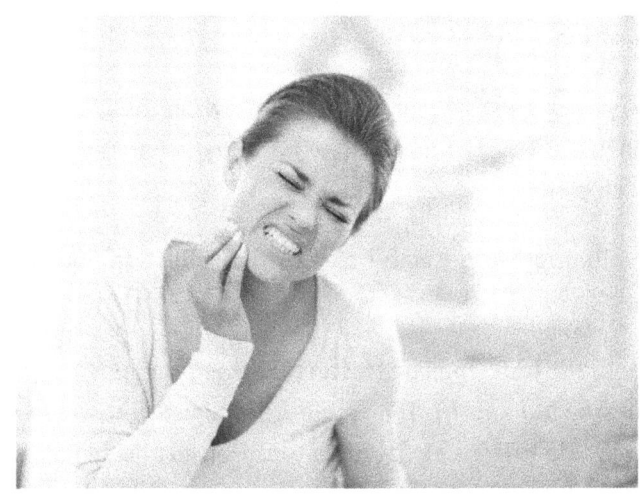

Some of the signs you experience can be symptomatic of other more serious ailments so it can be difficult to give an accurate diagnosis without the assistance of your dentist.

These are the general signs of toothache:

- Sharp, shooting acute pain isolated to the affected area that comes and goes (this could be caused by tooth sensitivity, head tension or stress as well as the tooth possibly being cracked or exposed to air.

- Dull throbbing chronic pain that lingers for a longer period of time.

The next symptoms are not as common. If you experience any of the following, please contact an emergency dentist as soon as possible:

- Are you experiencing fever?

- Are you finding breathing and swallowing difficult?

- Is the affected area surrounding the tooth swollen? is your check or jaw the same side as the affected area also swollen and feeling sensitive to the touch (almost like a tingling sensation?)

- Are your glands swollen under your jaw on the affected tooth's side? this usually means that the body is fighting an infection which exhibits as fever.

- Is your tooth too painful to eat, is it affecting your eating or sleeping?

- Is there a foul smelling, tasting discharge of pus coming from the affected tooth? This could be a sign of abscess infection which when left untreated can end up in the bloodstream. It can also spread to and infect the surrounding bone of the affected tooth.

These are signs of infection. Seek immediate medical attention if you are experiencing any of these, because if left untreated can lead to complications.

Chapter 4: Toothache Pain and What It Means

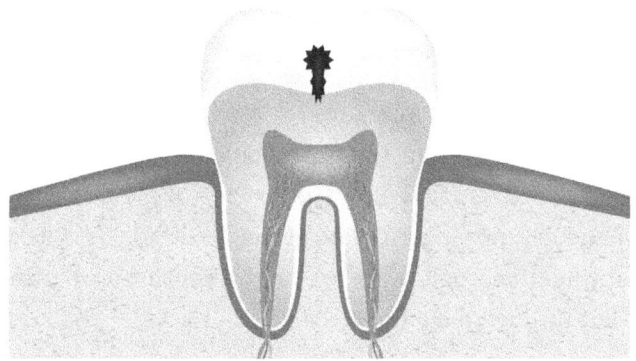

As we touched upon before, different types of tooth related pain can be an indicator of different problems.

Sharp, shooting pain:

Can indicate tooth sensitivity or hypersensitivity due to wear and tear and demineralization of tooth enamel from brushing (especially with a hard bristle brush), gum recession where the root is being exposed to more air than usual, decaying dental cavity, cracked tooth or abscess.

Chronic, lingering pain:

Suffering from this type of toothache could be the result of nerve damage from grinding the teeth, advanced tooth decay which has penetrated and damaged the nerve, trauma to the affected area through injury.

Pain or discomfort while eating:

Usually arises from tooth decay or a cracked tooth.

Severe throbbing pain:

Along with a swollen face or lymph nodes, swelling under the jaw of the affected side is usually an indicator of infection from an abscess.

Pain to the back of the jaw:

Particularly where the molars are situated may be due to impacted wisdom teeth where the teeth on some occasions only partially come through or remain below the surface of the gum line causing pain whenever applying pressure through biting. It's a pain similar to a baby teething only with the added tension of the teeth not able to cut through the gum.

This type of pain could also indicate TMJ (Temporomandibular Joint disorder) or Bruxism (tooth grinding), which can express pain in the jaw and in the facial bones such as the cheekbones and the boney structure within the outer ear canals.

You can feel this structure where the hinge is located linking the upper and lower jaws by simply inserting your index finger into your ear while chewing at the same time, that movement you experience is the Temporomandibular joint. This type of movement causes joint friction and discomfort for sufferers of TMJ.

Whatever the cause, your toothache could represent other problems. It's best to get this checked out by your dental professional while you treat the immediate pain now.

Chapter 5: Get Rid of a Toothache with Home Remedies

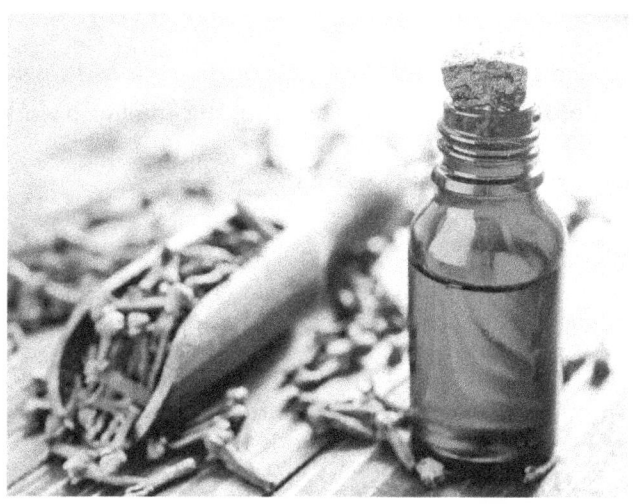

So here it is, twenty natural treatments that have been highly effective in the treatment of toothache pain while helping to reduce infection.

Some remedies outlined here offer relief within an hour while others take effect within a few hours of application. These remedies are for pain relief only and do not replace the need for a good dentist.

This should only be used as a temporary measure to help relieve pain if you are not able to get to a dentist immediately because there is no substitute for proper dental treatment that can get the real heart of the matter and treat the root cause (no pun intended) affecting your teeth which may be beyond the scope of just natural pain relief alone. Treating the cause rather than just treating the symptoms of pain is the best solution for permanent, pain free results.

There are several natural remedies using things you already have around your home that can provide pain relief for your toothache. Because these are natural they leave no known side effects and are easy to implement. There are a couple of treatments that pregnant women should avoid.

These remedies may seem like hocus pocus potions straight out of the pages of Hogwarts book of spells but they really do work.

Ice Compress and Ice Cold Mouth Rinse

Depending upon the type of toothache you have, for example if you have the toothache due to hypersensitivity then this might not be the best option for you. If you're not overly sensitive to cold then this may be an effective solution. Toothache arising from non sensitivity usually indicates infection where ice is the best line of defense.

Ice works by numbing the localized area by interrupting the pain signals the nerve cells transmit to the brain giving you temporary relief. It also reduces swelling and inflammation that arises from infection from abscesses.

These are several ways in which you can use ice to give pain relief, choose any one of the following:

Directions:

1. Wrap an ice cube inside a washcloth, run cold water over it for 10 seconds, enough to dampen the area containing the ice cube (this allows for the coolness of the ice cube to permeate through the washcloth). Place on the tooth itself or within the area of the toothache. This should help to take the edge off the pain.

2. Try using an icepack if you have one. This is also effective for numbing pain on the affected area. Place the icepack directly on the affected side and compress it. This should be applied to the cheek or jaw that is causing the most pain and discomfort.

   This should help to dull the pain within a few minutes. If you don't have an icepack, a Ziploc bag or a bag of frozen vegetables works as just as well.

3. Rubbing ice or an ice cube directly on the cheek over the area of pain gives almost instant pain relief.

4. Try placing an ice cube or a piece of ice in your mouth directly over the affected tooth or area of pain. Leave it in for as long as you can, until it completely melts is ideal. The longer you leave it in the greater the numbing effect on the pain.

5. Swirling and rinsing the mouth with cold water or ice water is effective at minimizing pain.

Salt Water Gargle

Salt has been used for over 3,500 years as a natural food preserve and for its ability to kill bacteria which is why salt is still recommended to this day for the natural treatment of wounds and infections and has been known to be highly effective in the treatment of toothache.

What makes salt such a great anti bacterial is that it draws water from bacteria through osmosis causing the bacteria shrink and die.

Osmosis is the process whereby water from a lower saline concentration travels across the cell membrane barrier to higher concentrations. The bacteria in the presence of high saline or salty environments are destroyed by dehydration which is why salt is such an effective preserve, from the time of the ancient Egyptians and was even used in the process of mummification.

Most toothaches arise from some kind of infection whether from a cracked tooth or missing filling, bacteria takes hold from food particles which have decomposed and are lodged within cavities where infection sets in.

Salt is ideal in the treatment of infection while addressing the issue of pain arising from the infected tooth. If you treat more than just the symptom of pain and treat the cause you will be able to eliminate the pain permanently.

Salt water has a two-fold purpose as it draws out infection from the affected gum tissue surrounding the nerve it kills bacteria while giving pain relief at the same time.

Directions:

Create a saline solution by simply adding a teaspoon of sea salt to a glass of lukewarm water and rinse around your mouth for around 20 to 30 seconds before spitting out. The saline solution cleans the area surrounding the tooth and helps draw out of some the infection responsible for the inflammation and pain. This treatment is safe and you can repeat as frequently as required until the pain subsides. You can also add sea salt or rock salt directly to the tooth or affected area if you don't mind the salty taste.

Sharp, intense pain should subside within a few minutes of treatment.

Acupressure (Not Recommended For Pregnant Women)

You have several different pressure points located all over your body, Ancient Chinese alternative medicine discovered that by simply applying pressure to these points can give pain relief, in particular if the correct pressure point associated with that pain is properly targeted.

Scientific studies have confirmed this theory and found that by applying adequate pressure to these points encourages the brain to release endorphins, the body's natural feel painkiller, directly to the site of pain.

There is a nerve situated in between the thumb and the index finger that shares the same pain receptors as the teeth. Applying ice on this pressure point interrupts the pain signal to the brain which relieves pain temporarily.

Use one or more of the following techniques:

Directions:

Place an ice cube on the part of the hand between the thumb and the index finger; in case you're not sure which part of the hand that is it's the webbed fleshy looking part of the hand. In the case of your left hand it's the part of the hand that forms an 'L' shape between the thumb and the forefinger. This pressure point has been known to influence tooth pain.

Hold the ice cube firmly in place on the "L" shaped part of the hand for at least 10 to 20 minutes, keeping it in the same spot until you start to experience pain relief.

For more severe toothache, create an ice bath by combining 2 cups of crushed ice to 2 cups of water into a medium sized bowl. Place your hand into the bowl while massaging the soft fleshy webbed part with your other hand. Do this for 1 minute at a time to avoid your hand getting too cold. This should alleviate pain within a few minutes.

Another technique is to grab the soft fleshy webbed part of your hand using your thumb and index finger. Apply pressure for between 2 and 3 minutes. This releases the body's endorphin, feel good hormones which is a great natural pain relief relying on the body's own abilities. Warning - Do not use this technique if pregnant.

Another acupressure point is located in the soft area of the Achilles tendon. Grasp this part of the ankle between the thumb and index finger applying pressure for 2 to 3 minutes.

Release and repeat.

Garlic Clove

Apart from warding off vampires, garlic has proven itself over the millennia as an effective antiseptic. Garlic has been recorded as far back as 3,000 BC for medicinal purposes and was used by the ancient Egyptians, the Romans and the Greeks which is why it is still so important in these cultures today.

Garlic contains Allicin, the compound responsible for its healing action making garlic a powerful antibacterial agent and a natural anesthetic. Allicin is released from the garlic once crushed giving pain relief to the affected area it is applied to.

Choose any of the following:

Directions:

1. Combine one clove of garlic with a sprinkling of rock salt and crush into a fine paste. Apply directly to the affected tooth but apply sparingly as too much can leave a burning sensation.

2. A clove of garlic crushed with a teaspoon of peanut butter applied to the tooth is also effective for pain relief.

3. You can also place a whole clove of garlic on the tooth for 30 minutes. If you're able to apply pressure, bite down on the clove allowing some of the juice to release on the affected tooth providing a natural soothing anesthetic. Gives relief within 20 minutes.

Chewing a clove of garlic also strengthens the immunity of the weakened tooth enabling it to heal from infection reducing pain and inflammation.

Onion

Like garlic, onion also has its share of miracle healing properties and is a natural antiseptic.

The early pioneers that settled in America used onions to treat asthma and colds. In China, onions were used to also treat coughs, congestion problems and bacterial infections. In fact so potent are the medicinal properties of the onion in the treatment of ailments that it has been officially recognized by the World Health Organization.

Directions:

Place a piece of onion big enough to cover the affected tooth. Leave on the tooth for 30 minutes to help kill bacteria and give pain relief.

If the tooth allows for it, cut off a bite sized piece of onion and chew it for two to three minutes. This will release the antiseptic qualities of the onion and help the pain to subside.

Pure Vanilla Extract and Almond Extract

Because pure Vanilla Extract and Almond Extract both contain alcohol (Vanilla extract has a slightly higher alcoholic content making it a little more effective than Almond extract), they both offer pain killing properties.

Directions:

Using either a cotton ball or a q-tip, soak with the pure vanilla extract solution and apply to the affected tooth or area. This should provide a numbing sensation within minutes.

Oats

Oats can be used to draw out pus and infection especially if an abscess is present.

Directions:

Place a teaspoon of oats onto the affected tooth and gently bite down. Leave for ten minutes before rinsing with a mixture of rock salt and water.

Iodine

From the early twentieth century Iodine has been used to disinfect drinking water from contaminated sources which makes Iodine such an effective topical treatment for open wounds exposed to bacteria.

Directions:

Place one drop of Iodine on the tooth, do not swallow it. Leave for 2 minutes; thoroughly rinse your mouth with water.

Hydrogen Peroxide (Food Grade)

Hydrogen Peroxide kills infection by altering bacteria's molecular structure. Through the process of oxidation Hydrogen Peroxide attacks bacteria by destabilizing its molecules causing them to break apart rendering them useless. This is why Hydrogen Peroxide foams upon contact with open wounds in the presence of bacteria.

You can get food grade hydrogen peroxide from your pharmacy.

Directions:

To receive pain relief using Hydrogen Peroxide, take a swig of three percent (food grade) Hydrogen Peroxide and swish around the mouth like mouth wash, spit it out and rinse thoroughly several times afterward with water.

You can also add half a glass of Hydrogen Peroxide (three percent food grade) to half a glass of water, swishing it around in your mouth for 30 seconds before spitting it out rinsing thoroughly with lukewarm salt water.

Pepper

Long considered a main fixture of the kitchen the world over and usually associated with adding flavor to food, Pepper can actually provide great pain relief from a toothache in addition to lessening the sensation of heightened tooth sensitivity.

Directions:

Add a quarter of a teaspoon of crushed rock salt to a pinch of pepper, mix well and place upon the sore tooth.

Brushing with this mixture on a daily basis provides protection against cavities, fights against bad breath and bleeding gums, cures tooth sensitivity and wards off toothache pain.

Ginger Root

Being indigenous to India and China, Ginger is highly regarded as one of the world's most important spices. For centuries it has been used for its flavor and for its curative properties, some of which include the aiding of digestion, lowering the levels of bad (LDL) cholesterol in the body and lowering blood pressure naturally by relaxing the constricting arterial walls which narrow with age and restrict normal blood flow.

Ginger is an extremely effective solution either in its raw or powdered form in the fight against toothache pain.

Powdered Ginger: Directions:

Place a teaspoon of powdered Ginger and Cayenne pepper into a cup and add a few drops of water, mix until it becomes a watery paste. Place a cotton ball into the mixture until it's saturated and place on the affected tooth. Try to keep the cotton ball on the tooth as the Cayenne pepper can irritate the surrounding gums.

Ginger without the Cayenne pepper is equally as effective in the relief of toothache pain just as is Cayenne pepper without the Ginger.

Raw Ginger: Directions:

You can purchase whole Ginger root at the grocery store and is effective for providing rapid toothache relief.

Cut an inch piece size of Ginger root, peel off the skin layer and place the piece of Ginger on the affected tooth. If able, gently bite down holding it in place. Doing this alone can rapidly decrease pain as the healing properties of the Ginger become absorbed into the surrounded affected area. Again, if you're able to do so, chew the piece of the Ginger swishing the Ginger juice around the painful tooth.

The remaining Ginger root should provide long term relief and can be stored in the refrigerator should you need additional treatment. The Ginger root also keeps well at room temperature as the cut part of the Ginger root forms a natural seal keeping it fresh for longer.

Vitamin D

People who suffer from Rickets have a vitamin D deficiency. The lack of vitamin D in the body contributes to weak bones which eventually affects the teeth.

These days milk is fortified by Vitamin D so that children can develop strong healthy bones.

Your body also manufactures its own Vitamin D in the presence of sunlight, in fact 20 to 30 minutes per day is enough to give your body the dose that it needs. This may not be the ideal solution for those who live in countries with low burn times where the risk of skin cancer is high, or in countries with low levels of sunlight or during times of winter. In these situations you can gain your dose of daily Vitamin D just by incorporating Vitamin D rich foods into your diet such as egg yolks, yoghurt, cream, butter and tuna fish. For vegans or vegetarians, Vitamin D also comes in the form of dietary supplements.

Vitamin D the old fashioned way, by exposing the gums and teeth to direct sunlight, no matter how funny you may look is actually beneficial because Ultra Violet light has bactericidal properties at wavelengths of 260 to 280 (nm) nanometers, killing off harmful bacteria infecting the teeth and gums. So effective is this method that dentists and hospitals use similar methods for sterilization today.

Clove and Clove Oil

Cloves have been revered for centuries for their antiseptic and anesthetic properties, both its fresh and dehydrated forms are effective in the relief of toothache pain.

The Clove has made several appearances throughout history and was used as far back as 200 BC in China for the relief of toothache pain and to freshen the breath. During the 19th century, long before the dental hygiene we know of today existed, the dentists of the time would carry liberal supplies of clove oil to numb their patient's mouths before and after extraction and for the alleviation of toothache pain. Clove oil is extracted from the clove bud which through its Eugenol content gains its bactericidal, anesthetic qualities making it an effective natural painkiller.

Cloves are still an effective way to manage toothache pain to this day and its longevity throughout the ages is proof of this.

Use any of the following methods:

Directions:

Place a fresh or dehydrated clove on the painful part of the tooth and bite down gently for thirty minutes, if the pain allows chew the clove until soft allowing the natural oil to permeate the affected area. If the pain persists, chew a second one. Because clove contains analgesic qualities you should experience numbness to the area within minutes of application.

You can also apply clove oil directly to the affected spot with a q-tip avoiding the tongue and surrounding gum area. In addition to having a strong, concentrated unpleasant taste of cloves, it can also irritate the surrounding tissue. Leaving on for 3 minutes should adequately numb the painful tooth.

Clove oil is for external use only and should not to be swallowed but rather rinsed thoroughly with water after application. More than 2 applications with clove oil is not recommended. Clove oil can be toxic if taken in large quantities.

Tea Tree Oil (Not Recommended For Pregnant Women)

Tea tree oil has long been hailed as a natural antiseptic by the native Aborigine's of the Australian outback, long before modern day science was able to confirm its medicinal properties.

The beauty of tea tree oil is its ability to penetrate, this means that it is ideal for deep treatment of the infected tissue affecting the tooth. Its antibacterial qualities kill infection while its painkilling and wound healing properties sooth and help repair the damaged tissue.

Directions:

Create a mouthwash by adding 3 drops of tea tree oil to 1 glass of water, stir well. Take a mouthful and swill it for 30 seconds at a time, spit out. Repeat again. Rinse the mouth thoroughly with a solution of lukewarm salt water. Do not swallow the tea tree oil mixture.

You should experience a noticeable dulling of the pain and a numbing sensation after the second mouthwash treatment; this is due to tea tree oil's penetrating properties which permeates the gum tissue to desensitize the nerves transmitting pain signals. The gums should also reduce in pain, redness and swelling as the tea tree kills the infection caused from bacteria.

Peppermint (Scientific name: Mentha Piperita)

Peppermint is another of nature's great anti-inflammatory elixirs, because of its menthol content it acts as a natural anesthetic and bactericide when applied directly to the area of pain. This is why menthol is an active ingredient in muscle and joint pain relief creams such as Deep Heat and Ben Gay. It's also used to alleviate cold and flu symptoms and is an effective decongestant. Peppermint also has a calming, soothing effect which is why it is so widely used in homeopathy and is considered an ideal remedy for toothache pain owing to its anesthetic qualities.

Directions:

Place four grams of fresh peppermint leaves into a coffee mug and fill it with boiling water. Add a teaspoon of salt and stir thoroughly. Allow the peppermint tea to cool until it is lukewarm, this ensures that the anesthetic properties permeate thoroughly into the tea, then drink. While drinking, swish the tea around in your mouth making sure you get good coverage over the area giving you pain, then swallow. After ten to fifteen minutes the pain should dull and subside.

Not only does this get to the heart of the toothache pain as it makes direct contact with the affected area but it also relieves pain internally too, much like how aspirin takes effect getting rid of the discomfort usually associated with toothache such as aching jaw, cheek and headache.

Dried Peppermint leaves

Peppermint doesn't have to be fresh for it to be effective, dried peppermint works just as well.

Directions:

Instead of making a tea, take the dried leaves and firmly pack them around the sore tooth, if you are able to apply pressure, gently bite down and hold for ten to twenty minutes. If you can, chew the leaves then spit out. Peppermint is excellent for drawing out any infection associated with toothache while acting as a natural painkiller.

Tea

Who would have thought the humble tea bag could provide such remarkable healing properties?

It was believed in ancient China that tea had curative abilities and that it was a major ingredient in the treatment of headache pain. It was then discovered that topical application also proved effective in the elimination of toothache pain. In addition to its soothing qualities, tea has been found to be an antibacterial, killing bacteria, viruses as well as fungi contained within the body. This makes it an ideal candidate in the treatment of toothache especially where infection is involved.

Due to the antioxidant properties which are derived from its polyphenols, tea is fast gaining popularity with scientists for its ability to fight against disease and for its protection against colon cancer and tumors.

Directions:

Place a standard teabag into a cup of water, place in the microwave for 1 minute. Remove the teabag while still warm and place on the sore tooth. Bite down gently and hold in place for 20 minutes or until you get pain relief.

Substituting green tea instead of regular tea works as equally well.

Wheatgrass

Wheatgrass is the juvenile stage in the lifecycle of wheat. It contains chlorophylls which are a natural antiseptic. Wheatgrass is quite remarkable in that it penetrates deep tissue to heal wounds and ulcers caused by infection by killing bacteria on affected sites while reducing pain and inflammation in the process, the perfect treatment for a painful tooth.

You can get live wheatgrass from your local health store or from your supermarket.

Directions:

Juice from wheat grass can be made into a mouthwash. Place a few good handfuls of wheatgrass into a fruit and vegetable juice extractor. Extract the juice. Take a mouthful of wheatgrass juice, undiluted and swill it in your mouth with greater focus given to the affected area. Hold in the mouth for at least 30 seconds before swallowing.

Taking wheatgrass internally has several health benefits. One major advantage of including wheatgrass in your diet is that it can prevent further tooth decay, addressing the heart of the pain in the first place.

If the taste proves too strong for you to swallow, you can spit it out.

In addition to extracting the juice of wheatgrass you can also break off the fresh shoots and chew them for a minute at a time. This also gets relief directly to the site of the pain.

Cucumber

Owing to its Vitamin C content in the form of ascorbic acid, Cucumber makes an effective anti-inflammatory and aides the reduction of swelling while drawing out bacterial infection.

Directions:

You can get cucumber from just about anywhere these days. Take one cucumber and slice off a half inch think piece. Bit down gently on the affected tooth and hold in place for 10 minutes. Easing of the pain should be experienced within that time period.

Refrigerating the cucumber helps to further reduce swelling and pain.

Covering

If your tooth has a large cavity or if the filling or the tooth is chipped or partially missing then being exposed to air will increase the chances of infection and pain. Food particles get into the cavity attracting bacteria and infection.

To reduce the pain experienced from exposed cavity, chew a piece of sugar free gum and gently press down, if able to do so, into the cavity. This creates a temporary seal preventing food from further collecting worsening infection. This protective seals also gives relief against sensitivity due to hot and cot fluids and aggravation from exposure to cold drafts.

Other individuals have reported relief from not only placing sugar free chewing gum over the cavity to crushed up aspirin (be careful with this one as direct contact to gums can cause a burning sensation), to pieces of garlic, cucumber and onion to placing extra strength Sensodyne toothpaste on the cavity to act as a temporary seal until a dentist visit is possible.

Avoid chewing food on the affected side if covering the exposed cavity.

Asafoetida (scientific name: Ferula foetida)

Asafoetida is extracted from the genus ferula plant and comes in the form of a resinous gum. Once the plant stems are cut, it oozes sap which solidifies into its resin form. It is used as a condiment to flavor curry dishes both in India and the Middle East and has been a regular staple of natural herbal medicines in India. Not only is it revered for its medicinal qualities such as in the aiding of digestion and freshening the breath but it has been highly regarded and favored in the treatment of toothache pain.

Directions:

You should be able to buy this from your local Indian spice emporium, spice shop or your local grocery store.

Add a teaspoon of Asafoetida in powder form to 5 drops of freshly squeezed lemon juice. Mix thoroughly until it creates a fine paste then heat in the microwave for 30 seconds.

Apply topically to the painful tooth using a q-tip. This should give rapid relief within a few minutes.

CHAPTER 6: TOOTHACHE PREVENTION

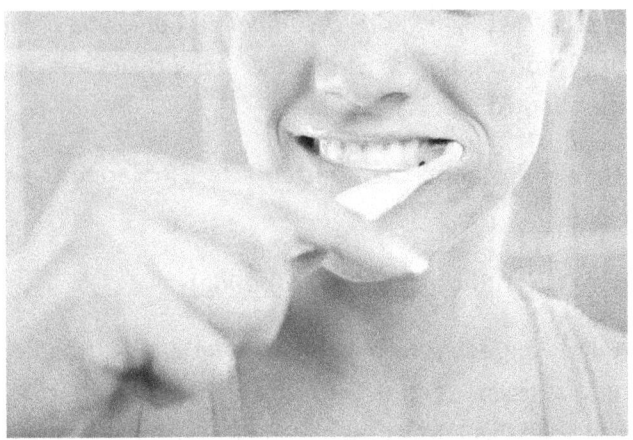

Having a toothache is no fun, the last thing you want to happen is to have another episode especially after what you experienced with this one.

To ensure that you prevent any future toothache or at the very least decrease the likelihood of it happening again there are preventative measures you can take.

First off, visit your dentist to get to the heart of the toothache in the first place, until the issue of the toothache is addressed and the problem treated, frequent toothache bouts are eminent.

Following the proper treatment there are changes to your lifestyle that can make a huge impact on the health of your teeth. In fact, the reason why you got the toothache in the first place was because your teeth were deteriorating as a result of diet and lifestyle and your tooth health was declining gradually on a daily basis. It wasn't even until you got the toothache that you realized that something was wrong yet it was a problem quietly building.

This is why they call tooth decay and gum disease the "Silent Killer", it accumulates over time and slowly creeps up on you.

By altering your diet you can greatly improve the condition and health of your teeth. For example just by simply adding more calcium and phosphate to your diet can actually reverse your teeth's enamel erosion by re-mineralizing them. The teeth are resilient creations and prior to reading this, most people aren't aware of this fact that your teeth have the ability to repair and rebuild themselves.

Most dentists won't even tell you this as they treat the solution of the toothache without arming you with the appropriate preventative measures you need to further preserve your teeth (other than the usual advice of proper brushing and flossing). In fact teeth don't have to weaken with age they can actually get stronger.

What kinds of foods contain recommended levels of calcium and phosphate?

You can find calcium in the more obvious sources such as milk, yogurt, cheese but you can also find them in chickpeas, tofu, nuts, oats, cabbage, broccoli, oranges, turnips, etc.

You need around 1,000 mg of calcium per day if you're aged between nineteen and fifty years of age, which you should get by having a good mixture of these types of calcium rich foods in a day. In fact having two yogurts and a cup of skim milk per day gives you around 1,100 mg a day, easily fulfilling your recommended daily requirement.

Phosphate you'll find from such foods as egg yolk, milk, nuts, beans, lentils, wheat germ, soy, oats, and corn. The great thing is that these foods are also a great source of calcium so you don't need to double up on your intake as you get a good dose of each from eating the same amount.

Brush with baking soda and avoid toothpastes that contain glycerin as this inhibits the tooth's natural ability to re-mineralize itself. Baking soda is effective at decreasing the amount of tooth eroding bacteria present in the mouth.

Avoid foods that are high in processed and refined flours and sugars. These attract tooth deteriorating bacteria which can damage your teeth on a daily basis and undo the re- mineralization process you're trying to achieve.

This is why our teeth are constantly eroded because the food we eat does not give them adequate time to heal and rebuild themselves.

Incorporate more fruits, vegetables and wholegrain breads into your diet. Vegetables and wholegrain breads introduce fiber which provides bulk and texture for cleaning plaque and bacteria off teeth.

Vitamin D as we spoke of earlier which fortifies and strengthens teeth from the inside out, you can get this naturally from sun exposure or from your diet in the form of fish oils such as found in salmon, tuna, cheese, egg yolks. Vitamin D aids in calcium absorption.

Change you toothbrush every 6 months or less. With wear and tear your toothbrush's bristles become less effective at sweeping plaque from around the gum line preventing gum disease.

Brush your teeth twice a day, preferably following a meal.

Floss your teeth daily, especially before bed; this minimizes the amount of bacteria-causing plaque that erodes your teeth while you sleep. When flossing it's not enough to floss in between teeth to prevent gingivitis, floss a little under the gum line. Food and bacteria that collect here is what contributes to periodontal disease, abscesses, gum recession and eventually tooth loss.

You'll want to get into a solid habit of flossing, you'll find that if you had gums that were sensitive or bled easily, with frequent flossing, the bleeding will cease, the gums will heal and will turn from red to a healthy pink color, which is the color gums should be.

Don't buy hard bristle toothbrushes, manufacturers should discontinue the hard bristle brush as it deteriorates the gums by pulling them away from the tooth which accelerates recession of the gum line.

Brush your tongue, lots of bacteria congregate and are deposited within the pores of the tongue causing bad breath. Bacteria coated tongues contribute to sore throat as scientists have found the tongue to be a breeding ground for harmful bacteria such as Streptococcus.

Chew sugar free gum after your last meal for the day, only one piece. Chewing gum throughout the entire day can cause flatulence and an excess of gum intake can cause explosive diarrhea due to the sugar substitute, Sorbitol. Just one piece after your last meal for the day produces saliva which is the body's natural defense in neutralizing bacteria.

Avoiding eating in between meals, this gives bacteria a chance to re-grow and erode the teeth. The bacteria can only live off the food you feed it which makes sugary snacks a no- no. If you feel peckish, have an apple or carrot sticks, this will ensure that your teeth remain clean as they provide bulk for cleaning the teeth while you eat.

Following these steps will not only decrease the risk of suffering a toothache again but also strengthen your teeth, gums and bones that will ensure that you keep your teeth long into the future.

Chapter 7: Conclusion

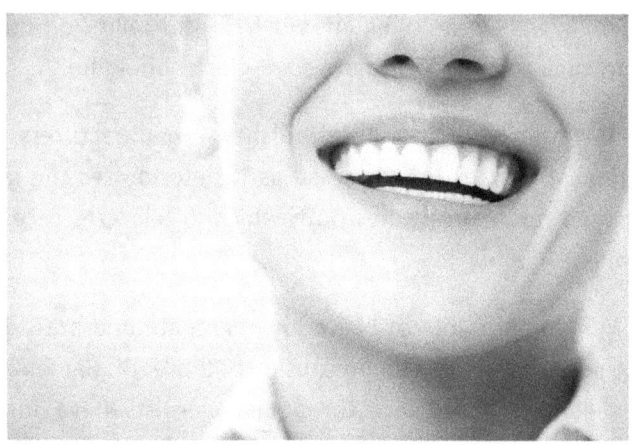

Tooth loss doesn't have to be a fact of life; you don't have to accept that it's inevitable with age.

There are still cultures in remote areas of the world that don't have access to the refined foods that we do or to proper dental treatment, yet they live their entire lives with their adult teeth intact and in perfect health.

We are meant to have teeth for a lifetime not just until our forty's and fifty's. As you've seen, it is possible to heal and strengthen your teeth from the inside out because they are living tissue and because of this fact, they can be repaired.

The best remedies come straight out of nature's own kitchen, the best methods that were discovered thousands of years ago still work today.

If you think about it, a toothache unless derived from a traumatic event took a while to build, our lack of immunity due to our poor diet and our current stressful lifestyle all play a part in the deterioration of our teeth.

Relying on natural solutions is beneficial for the body however if your tooth is abscessed and infected and the pain has spread to the jaw and lymph nodes, you must see a dentist as it can develop into a life threatening situation if not treated. Future prevention and by being vigilant is the key to a long life free of toothache pain.

So there you have it, twenty of the most potent natural toothache remedies that are all within your reach and the best part is, they are all natural, all work in their own right and have brought relief to the thousands that have used them the world over.

MEET THE AUTHOR

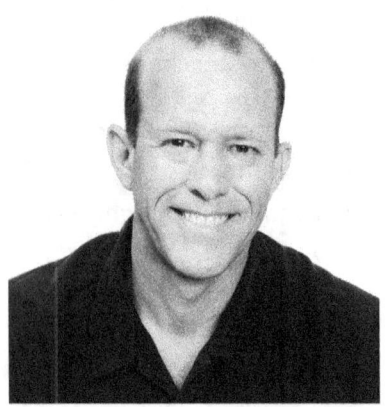

Hayden Anderson has a passion for helping others obtain peace and wellness. Sometimes that means changing lifestyle habits and addressing medical complexities through nutrition and alternative medicine. Hayden has years of experience in the area of holistic health, yoga, and meditation. He uses his experience and knowledge to change people's perception of eastern medicine.

As a kid Hayden suffered from a chronic illness that doctor's treated with medication. Hayden's parents were satisfied with doctor's maintaining his condition but Hayden wanted more. At nineteen Hayden became obsessed with eastern medicine and took control of his health. Through the use of herbs and dietary changes to complement his blood type, he was able throw away prescription medication that he had taken daily for as long as he could remember. He never looked back and is passionate about sharing his knowledge with others.

Hayden, his wife and kids enjoy spending time outdoors, growing their own food and herbs, sharing their day with each other around the family dinner table and game nights with old fashioned board games like Parcheesi, Aggravation, Sorry, Clue and Life.

MORE BOOKS BY HAYDEN ANDERSON

Irritable Bowel Syndrome: IBS Symptoms, Remedies and Prevention

Sleep Apnea: The Ultimate Guide on Diagnosing and Treating Sleep Apnea

www.ingramcontent.com/pod-product-compliance
Lightning Source LLC
LaVergne TN
LVHW021742060526
838200LV00052B/3420